17 Day Di Reloaded:

Delicious Cycle 1 Recipes Cookbook

For Your Rapid Weight Loss

By: Samantha Michaels

TABLE OF CONTENTS

Samantha Michaels

PUBLISHERS NOTES

Disclaimer

INTRODUCTION

The 17 Day Diet is made up four Cycles which aim to promote fast and healthy weight loss through these four core ideas:

- Accelerate,
- Activate,
- Achieve, and
- Arrive.

Each Cycle lasts for 17 days, during which a person is given a list of approved foods that he or she must strictly adhere to for the success of the program. The secret of this program lies on what is known as body confusion that is achieved through the changing food patterns throughout the four Cycles. This body confusion is a way of preventing the body from adapting to the metabolic properties that allow you to burn more fat faster.

Cycle 1 is the initial 17-day period that will keep you away from all the starchy foods, sugars, and carbohydrates that you know and love. It is considered to be the strictest of all the cycles, but also allows the most weight loss as it cleanses the body of unhealthy carbs that result to all those extra pounds. Furthermore, this cycle stimulates the body's metabolic rate, allowing it to burn up fat and calories faster.

The good thing about this first cycle is that while you may be deprived of all the pasta, breads, and sweets that you have grown to want and love, it does allow you to eat unlimited amounts of certain proteins and vegetables, keeping you from depriving your body of the nutrients that it needs. Here is a list of some of the most delicious recipes that you can try out during your Cycle 1 period.

CHAPTER 1 - BREAKFAST RECIPES

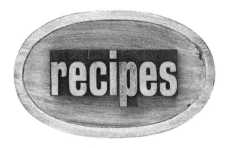

Breakfast Bowl

This breakfast treat is easy to do and very filling. Most of the ingredients are already those that you may have on hand, so it is not easy to prepare either.

Ingredients:

¼ cup Ground Turkey
¼ cup Mushrooms
¼ cup Bell Peppers (sliced and frozen)
¼ cup Roasted Bell Peppers
2 pcs. Egg whites
¼ cup Mozzarella, shredded

Procedure:

Prepare all the ingredients and keep the handy and ready to use.
In a medium-sized pan, heat about 1tablespoon of vegetable oil.
Sautee the mushrooms and bell-peppers, and add in the turkey sausage.
When the meat is tender, add the egg whites and stir until cooked.
Season with salt and pepper to your preferred taste.
Transfer to a plate, sprinkle with shredded mozzarella cheese.

Enjoy!

You can also change or add vegetables such as substituting tomatoes for the bell-peppers and adding onions to the recipe. The good thing about this recipe is you can practically use whatever vegetable you have and come up with a healthy egg-white omelets that will give you the energy to start your day.

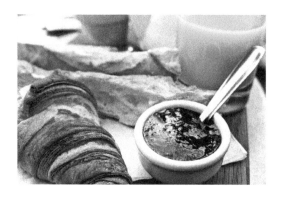

Mock French Toast

French toast has always been a breakfast favourite for many people, and with this recipe, you can have it and still stick to your diet as well. For this breakfast treat, all you need are 2 simple ingredients and some flavouring for taste. This recipe is also sometimes referred to as apple pancakes.

Ingredients:

1 Apple
1 pc Whole Egg or 2pcs Egg whites
*cinnamon or vanilla to taste

Procedure:

Spray some oil onto a skillet or put just enough oil to coat the bottom of the pan, and then turn the heat on to medium.

Samantha Michaels

Slice the apples into thin pieces. Make sure to remove the core or the seeds.

When the pan is hot, lay the apples on the bottom of the pan so that no apples are overlapping.

Cover the pan, lower the heat, and cook for about 2minutes or until the apple slices are softened.

Meanwhile, whisk your egg or egg whites and add about a teaspoon of cinnamon and 1/4teaspoon vanilla. Mix well.

Pour the egg mixture over the apples and let all the egg cook. Try to lift the parts that are already cooked to let the raw egg flow to the bottom of the pan to be cooked.

When there is no more liquid egg left, cover the pan and cook for another 2minutes.

Flip the eggs onto the other side. Cover and cook again for another minute or so.

Slide onto your plate. Enjoy!

For an added treat, top off with fat-free yogurt. Truly yummy and satisfying!

Baked Apple Tarts

This is very similar to the Mock French Toast, with the only difference being in the cooking method used. If you have more time on your hands or if you would rather just leave the cooking to your oven, this recipe should be just right for you.

Ingredients:

1 pc Apple, cored and thinly sliced
1 pc Egg or 2 pcs Egg whites
1 teaspoon Cinnamon
¼ teaspoon Vanilla

Procedure:

Pre-heat your oven to 375°F.

In a baking pan, line the thin slices of apple so that they cover the bottom of the pan.

Whisk the eggs with the cinnamon and vanilla, and pour over the apples.

Bake for about five minutes or until the apples are soft and the egg is cooked through.

Serve and enjoy.

You can also use a microwave-safe dish and cook this in the microwave for about 2-3minutes. This is a good way to satisfy your sweet tooth too.

Favorite Breakfast

This recipe is fairly easy to do, and can easily be done ahead of time for that quick and satisfying breakfast. It is really filling as well and packs a lot of vegetables for a really healthy dish.

Ingredients:

5 cups Fresh Baby Spinach
6 large pcs Mushrooms
4 large pcs Tomatoes
1/3 cup Onions, chopped
2-3 cloves Garlic, minced
White wine vinegar or Balsamic vinegar
Salt and Pepper to taste
2 Tablespoons Olive Oil

Procedure:

Prepare your ingredients. Slice the mushrooms, tomatoes, and onions. Mince the garlic and chop the fresh baby spinach. Prepare a bow to fit all ingredients later.

Heat some of the olive oil in a pan, then sauté the mushrooms and set aside in the bowl.

Next, sauté the onions, add the garlic, and sauté the tomatoes as well. Set aside with the mushrooms.

Pour in all of the remaining olive oil onto the pan and sauté the baby spinach until cooked.

Carefully stir in all the other ingredients back into the pan with the baby spinach.

Add a splash of vinegar, about 1 tablespoon or so.

Sprinkle with salt and pepper to taste.

Transfer to plate and serve.

For a more filling meal, get a portion of the vegetables and mix with scrambled eggs. Also makes a great snack! You can store in an airtight container and keep in the freezer until ready to cook.

Feta and Spinach Egg Omelette

You can never have enough eggs when you're in cycle 1. The good thing is, eggs are so versatile that you can cook them up with almost anything you want so that you never get tired of it. Here is a simple scrambled egg recipe that uses feta cheese for that slightly salty and tangy flavour.

Ingredients:

1 Egg or 2pcs Egg whites
1 cup Spinach, chopped
¼ cup Feta cheese, grated

Procedure:

Spray a cooking pan with some oil, or pour a little amount just enough to grease the bottom of the pan.

Whish the eggs, add the chopped spinach and the grated feta cheese.

Pour egg mixture onto pan and cook at medium heat until there is no more liquid egg left.

Serve onto plate. Enjoy!

You can also add some cooked Tempeh bacon for additional flavour. Tempeh is an approved probiotic for cycle 1 that can be bought in most whole foods and vegetarian stores.

Greek Eggs Level Up

Greek eggs are typically scrambled eggs with feta cheese. Because of the salty taste of the cheese, there is no need to add any additional seasoning. Here is a recipe that adds a bit more kick to the classic dish, and it will definitely help you put a fresh start to your day.

Ingredients:

2 Whole Eggs or 4pcs Egg whites
2 Tablespoons Feta Cheese, fat-free
¼ cup Tomatoes
¼ cup Bell peppers
1/8 tsp. Salt
Green Onions
Cumin
Lemon Juice

Procedure:

Cut up the tomatoes, bell peppers and green onions.
Scramble the eggs. Mix in the vegetables.
Tear up the feta cheese into pieces and mix into the egg mixture.
Season with a pinch or two of cumin, depending if you like it hot, then add a splash of lemon juice.
Spray a pan with some oil, just until the bottom is greased, then put over medium heat.

Samantha Michaels

When the pan is hot, pour in the scrambled egg and cook until preferred doneness. Make sure that there is no more liquid in the eggs.
Serve on a plate and enjoy!

You can adjust the seasoning depending on your taste. Either add more cumin or extra spices, or just remove them altogether. By doing so, you can enjoy this dish but make it a different taste every time.

Mushroom, Cheese, and Green Pepper Omelette

Just what the name says: an omelette filled with mushrooms, cheese, and green peppers. A perfect way to start your day!

Ingredients:

½ cup Mushrooms, chopped
½ Onion, minced
1 oz. Fat-free Cheddar Cheese, thinly sliced
¼ Green Bell pepper, chopped
2 Eggs
1 tablespoon Olive Oil
*Salt and Pepper to taste

Procedure:

Pour olive oil in a skillet over medium heat.
Sauté the onions, add the mushrooms, and then the green pepper.
Meanwhile, whisk the eggs and season with salt and pepper.
Add the cheese slices onto the skillet and then pour the egg over all the other ingredients.
Fry the omelette for about two minutes before flipping over to cook the other side.
Serve on a plate and enjoy!

Make sure that the egg is cooked all the way through and don't worry if it breaks when you try to flip it. This recipe is still guaranteed to taste great!

CHAPTER 2- MAIN ENTREES- CHICKEN DISHES

Chicken Breast

This dish is very easy to do, straightforward, and still makes up a satisfying meal. The ingredients are also what you would have on hand so preparing it would be a breeze.

Ingredients:

Chicken Breast
1 whole Onion, chopped
1 tablespoon Olive Oil
½ cup Water
Salt and Pepper to taste

Procedure:

Season the chicken breast with salt and pepper.
Prepare a grilling pan over medium heat, put 1 tablespoon of olive oil.
When the pan is hot, put the chicken in, add the chopped onions, and pour half a cup of water over the chicken.
Cook for about 20minutes or until the chicken is tender and cooked through.
Serve.

You can also bake this in a 400°F oven for thirty minutes or until golden brown in color. Yummy and healthy!

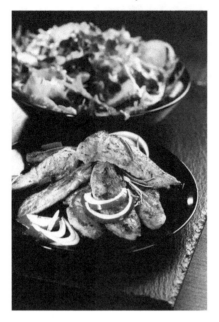

Balsamic Chicken Breasts

Here is a dish that makes use of a simple but flavourful marinade which can be made in just a few minutes. Perfect for chicken breasts, the marinade can also be used for other white meats such as fish.

Ingredients:

½ cup Balsamic Vinegar
1 tablespoon Olive oil
1 tablespoon Rosemary, chopped
1 clove Garlic, minced
½ teaspoon Salt
¼ teaspoon Pepper
4 pcs Boneless Chicken Breasts, skin removed

Procedure:

Create marinade. Combine vinegar, olive oil, rosemary, garlic, salt and pepper in a bowl.

Soak chicken breasts into marinade. Marinate for at least 30minutes.

Grill chicken breasts for about 8minutes on each side or bake at 350°F for 20-30minutes or until completely cooked through.

Transfer onto plate and enjoy!

You can also prepare this dish ahead of time and leave the chicken in the marinade overnight for a stronger flavour.

Balsamic Mustard Chicken Breast

Here is another easy marinade for a tasty chicken breast recipe! If you think that chicken breasts are bland and dry, try this recipe with balsamic vinegar and mustard and you may just change your mind.

Ingredients:

3 tablespoons Balsamic Vinegar
2 tablespoons Dijon Mustard
½ teaspoon Garlic, minced
1pc. Chicken Breast

Procedure:

Combine the vinegar, mustard, and minced garlic to create the marinade.

Coat the chicken in the marinade for at least 30 minutes. The longer you marinate the chicken, the better.

When ready to cook, heat a non-stick pan on medium heat. Place the chicken on the pan and pour the remaining marinade over the chicken.

Cook on each side for about 5 minutes or until slightly browned.

Serve on plate and enjoy!

You can adjust the ingredients according to your preferred taste. If the marinade dries out during cooking, you can add a little more vinegar to avoid the chicken from becoming dry. You can also add some sliced onions and mushrooms for added taste and texture. Also, try to make this ahead of time to let the chicken soak in the marinade longer.

Parmesan Chicken

A simple chicken recipe added with a cheesy twist! This is a great way to serve chicken in a different style.

Ingredients:

1lb. Chicken Breast
2 Eggs or 4 Egg Whites
4 tablespoons Water
2 tablespoons Olive Oil
¼-1/2 cup Parmesan Cheese, fat-free
1 teaspoon Garlic Powder
*Salt and Pepper to taste

Procedure:

Mix the dry ingredients: parmesan cheese, garlic powder, and salt and pepper in a bowl or zip lock bag.
Cut the chicken into strips or chunks, whichever you prefer.
Beat the eggs with the water.
Dip the chicken pieces in the egg before putting in the seasoning bag or bowl.
Shake the chicken to coat all pieces with the seasoning.
In a pan over medium heat, put the olive oil.
Cook the chicken in the pan until golden brown.
Transfer to plate. Enjoy!

Make sure to use fat-free parmesan cheese. You can also bake this dish at 350°F for a healthier alternative.

Chicken Stir Fry

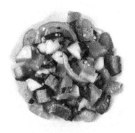

Stir fries are great meals to make. They are complete with meat and vegetables, easy to cook, and very tasty and flavourful. Here is a simple stir fry recipe that is perfect for your Cycle 1 diet.

Ingredients:

½ cup Broccoli, chopped
1pc. Carrot, cut into strips
1 whole Onion, chopped
1pc. Chicken Breast
*Salt and Pepper to taste

Procedure:

Prepare the ingredients. Chop the broccoli, cut the carrots into thin strips, chop the onion, and cut the chicken breast into strips or cubes.

Heat a non-stick pan over medium heat. When the pan is hot enough, toss in the onions and add the carrots and the broccoli. Cook until the carrots are a bit tender. Set aside in a bowl.

Put the chicken into the pan. Cover and let cook for about 10minutes, stirring occasionally to make sure that the chicken is cooked all the way through.

When the chicken is cooked, mix the vegetables back into the pan, sprinkle with salt and pepper to taste, and cook for another minute or two.

Serve on a plate and enjoy.

For added flavour, you can add a splash of light soy sauce into your stir fry while the vegetables and chicken are cooking. Make sure to let the chicken and vegetables absorb the liquid for a more flavourful chicken stir fry. You can also add mushrooms and other vegetables that you may have on hand.

Chicken with Mushrooms and Onions

This is a simple marinated chicken that is topped off with mushrooms and onions. Very simple to make but is a great dish even for those who are not on a diet.

Ingredients:

2pcs. Chicken Breasts
1 teaspoon Olive Oil
1 Lemon, juiced
2 cloves Garlic, minced
½ teaspoon Black Pepper
½ cup Water
1pc Onion, chopped
½ cup Mushrooms
2 tablespoons Light Soy Sauce

Procedure:

Combine the olive oil, lemon juice, minced garlic, and black pepper in a zip lock bag.

Samantha Michaels

Cut the chicken into strips or chunks. Put into the zip lock bag and marinate for 30minutes or more.

When ready to cook, heat a non-stick pan over medium heat and toss in the chicken and all of the marinade into the pan. Cook for 8-10minutes, stirring occasionally. When the chicken pieces are cooked all the way through, transfer to a plate and cover to keep it from cooling. Do not turn off the heat.

Pour half a cup of water into the pan, and then toss in the onions and the mushroom. Sautee until the onion becomes soft and the mushrooms release their moisture.

Season with salt and pepper, and then add the 2 tablespoons of light soy sauce.

Top the chicken with the mushrooms and onions. Enjoy!

Devilled Chicken

Chicken is a very versatile meat and can fit with almost any seasoning to satisfy all palates. If you like your chicken a bit on the spicy side, then this recipe is just for you.

Ingredients:

4pcs Chicken Breasts
1 tablespoon Olive Oil
1 tablespoon Apple Cider Vinegar
1 tablespoon Yellow Mustard
½ teaspoon Cayenne Pepper

Procedure:

Mix the olive oil, apple cider vinegar, yellow mustard and cayenne pepper in a bowl.
Rub the mixture onto the chicken breasts and marinate for at least 30minutes.
Pre-heat the oven to 375°F.

When the chicken has been marinated and the oven is at the desired temperature, bake the chicken for 40 minutes or until the chicken is tender.
Transfer to a plate and enjoy.

If you want to adjust the spice, simply modify the amount of cayenne pepper in the recipe. You can also grill the chicken and brush with the marinade while doing so to keep the chicken from being too dry.

Greek Chicken Patties

Chicken patties can taste as good as if not better than the regular beef patties that many people are used to. With the addition of some feta cheese, roasted tomatoes, and some fresh baby spinach, this dish will make you re-think what a burger patty should be like.

Ingredients:

1 kilo Ground Chicken
1 pack, Fresh Baby Spinach
½ cup Roasted Tomatoes, chopped
3 cloves Garlic, crushed
½ cup Red Onion, chopped
¼-½ cup Fat-free Feta Cheese
Pepper to taste

Procedure:

In a non-stick pan, sauté baby spinach until soft. Set aside and chop into small pieces.
Sauté the onion and garlic, then add to the baby spinach.
Add the chopped roasted tomatoes, and then add the ground chicken when the spinach and onion and garlic have cooled down.
Sprinkle some pepper to taste.

Samantha Michaels

When the chicken has been combined well with the other ingredients, mix in the chopped feta cheese.

Create small patties by rounding even potions into a ball and flattening the meat.

Cook the patties on the non-stick pan for about 3minutes on each side, or until the patty has cooked through.

Serve on a plate and enjoy!

You can store the patties in the freezer for future use. This is also great with a serving of fresh salad on the side. Yummy!

Grilled Balsamic Chicken

Here is another chicken marinade that is sure to be a favourite. Balsamic vinegar and mustards are used to create a slightly tangy, spicy flavour, while the Worcestershire sauce balances it all out to make a delectable dish. Prepare this recipe ahead of time to get the best results.

Ingredients:

6pcs Boneless Chicken Breasts, halved
¼ cup Fat-free Chicken Broth
½ cup Balsamic Vinegar
1/3 cup Scallion, chopped
2 tablespoons Dijon Mustard
1 tablespoon Garlic, minced
1 tablespoon Truvia Sweetener
2 teaspoons Worcestershire Sauce
1 teaspoon Dry Mustard
1 teaspoon Cracked Black Pepper

Procedure:

Combine the chicken broth, balsamic vinegar, chopped scallions, Dijon mustard, minced garlic, Truvia sweetener, Worcestershire sauce, dry mustard, and cracked black pepper in a large zip lock bag. Make sure that the bag is big enough for you to put in the chicken breasts as well.

Mix all the ingredients well to create the marinade.

Place the chicken in the zip lock bag and seal.

Store in the refrigerator and let the chicken marinate overnight. Make sure to turn it over occasionally to make sure that all parts of the chicken breasts are coated nicely.

When ready to cook, prepare your grill.

Grill the chicken for about 5minutes on each side or until golden brown in color. Make sure to brush with the marinade from time to time so that the chicken does not dry out.

Serve and enjoy!

Lemon Chicken

This is an easy chicken recipe that makes use of chicken broth, a lemon, rosemary, and some pepper. Yup, all the ingredients you need are simple to have, and the dish is even simpler to prepare. There is also no need to marinade the chicken for a long time so this is an excellent dish to make for when you are just tired and hungry from a long day at work.

Ingredients:

1 tablespoon Olive Oil
2pcs Chicken Breasts, halved
1 cup Low Sodium Chicken Broth
1pc. Lemon, zested and juiced
1 teaspoon Rosemary
*Ground Pepper to taste

Procedure:

Heat the olive oil in a pan over medium heat.

Cook the chicken on the pan for about 4minutes on each side or until slightly browned.

Meanwhile, mix all the other ingredients in a bowl: Pour in the chicken broth, add the lemon zest and the lemon juice, mix in 1 teaspoon of rosemary and a pinch or two of ground black pepper. Mix well.

When the chicken has been browned on both sides, pour the lemon mixture over the chicken and cover the pan. Let the chicken cook for another 30minutes or until the chicken is cooked through. Serve on a plate, enjoy!

You can substitute the rosemary for other herbs such as thyme or basil, whichever you prefer. The best thing about this recipe is that it is easy to do and it also gives you time for other things as well.

Sesame Chicken Stir Fry

Here is another chicken recipe that is easy to prepare and to cook. Stir fries are always a great way to combine simple ingredients and turn them into a meal that is truly satisfying. Did I mention how easy it is to do this recipe?

Ingredients:

1 pc. Chicken Breast, cut into chunks
1 small Red Bell pepper
1 teaspoon Garlic powder
¼ cup Mushrooms
¼ cup Fresh Green Beans
¼ cup Low Sodium Light Soy Sauce
2 teaspoons Olive Oil
1 tablespoon Sesame Seeds

Procedure:

In a pan over medium heat, place the chicken chunks and pour in the light soy sauce and olive oil. Stir occasionally and let cook until the chicken pieces are browned.

Chop all the vegetable ingredients and add to the chicken.

Sprinkle in the garlic powder and add the sesame seeds, then sauté until the vegetables are lightly cooked.

Serve and enjoy.

Oregano Chicken

You can never have too much chicken for your Cycle 1 period. The good thing is that there are a great number of ways on how to cook chicken and not let it taste the same way over and over again. This simple recipe makes use of seasonings that are already available in most homes.

Ingredients:

2 pcs. Chicken Breasts, de-boned and with skin removed
2 tablespoons Olive Oil
2 tablespoons Lemon Juice
1 tablespoon Worcestershire Sauce
1 tablespoon Low Sodium Soy Sauce
1 teaspoon Dried Oregano Leaves
½ teaspoon Garlic Powder
2 cloves Garlic, minced
*Salt and Pepper to taste

Procedure:

Combine the olive oil, lemon juice, Worcestershire sauce, soy sauce, oregano leaves, garlic powder, and minced garlic in a bowl and mix.

Season the chicken with salt and pepper and lay the pieces on an oven proof dish.

Pour the olive oil mixture over the chicken, cover, and let it marinate for 30minutes or more. Make sure to turn the chicken pieces occasionally to coat all sides properly.

Pre-heat the oven to 375°F.

When the oven is heated up, bake the chicken for 15minutes. Turn the chicken pieces onto the other side and bake for another 15minutes or until the chicken is cooked through.

Serve the chicken on a plate and pour the remaining sauce over it or into a separate bowl.

Enjoy.

Baked Parmesan Chicken

This chicken recipe is a real gourmet treat! You can serve it during parties or for special occasions, and it lets you stick to your diet too.

Ingredients:

1 lb. Chicken Breast, cut into strips or chunks
½ cup Fat-free Parmesan Cheese
½ teaspoon Salt
¼ teaspoon Pepper
¼ teaspoon Garlic Powder
½ tablespoon Basil
1 cup Sugar-free Marinara Sauce
½ cup Fat-free Mozzarella

Procedure:

In a zip lock bag, combine half cup parmesan cheese, salt, pepper, garlic powder, and basil.

Mix the chicken chunks or strips into the dry ingredients and shake well to coat all pieces.

Pre-heat the oven to 350°F.

Transfer the chicken to an oven-proof dish and top with 1cup of sugar-free marinara sauce.

Top with half cup of fat-free mozzarella.

Cover with foil and bake for 30minutes or until chicken is cooked through.

Serve and enjoy!

Twice-cooked Chicken

While this dish may require a little more effort than most recipes, it is sure to be tender, tasty, and an all-time favourite.

Ingredients:

1 tablespoon Olive Oil
3pcs Chicken Breasts, de-boned and skins removed
½ pc. Onion
6 pcs. Large Mushrooms

Procedure:

Cook the chicken in a non-stick pan over medium heat until lightly browned. Transfer the chicken to an oven-safe dish and set aside.

Meanwhile, pre-heat the oven to 325°F, slice the onions and the mushrooms.

Sauté the onions and the mushrooms in the pan in which the chicken was cooked; this will take about 3-4 minutes

Spoon the onions and the mushrooms over the chicken then cover with foil.

Bake in the pre-heated oven for 45 minutes or until the chicken is cooked all the way through.

Serve onto plates and enjoy!

Stuffed Chicken Breasts

Chicken with a secret surprise inside. A real treat!

Samantha Michaels

Ingredients:

4 pcs Chicken Breasts
4 oz. Fat-free Cottage Cheese
3 tablespoons Spinach, diced
1 teaspoon Garlic Powder
1 teaspoon Onion Powder
1 tablespoon Parmesan Cheese
1 teaspoon Black Pepper

Procedure:

Pound the chicken breasts and flatten nicely.
Mix the cottage cheese, chopped onions, diced spinach, garlic powder, and black pepper.
Place about 3spoonfuls of the cheese mixture at the center of two of the chicken breasts, and then cover each with the remaining chicken breasts. You can use toothpicks to hold the chicken pieces together.
Pre-heat the oven to 400°F
Place the stuffed chicken in an oven-proof dish and bake in the pre-heated oven for 35-40minutes.
Enjoy!

CHAPTER 3- MAIN ENTREES- TURKEY DISHES

Stuffed Turkey Patties

Here is a turkey recipe that will give you a break from all those chicken dishes for your diet program. Turkey patties are stuffed with onion and cheese to keep it flavourful and tasty.

Ingredients:

1 lb. Ground Turkey
1 Onion, diced
½ cup Fat-free Feta Cheese
1 teaspoon Olive Oil

Procedure:

Dice the onion and cut the fat-free feta cheese into small pieces.
Divide the ground turkey into 3 equal portions.
Flatten one portion of the ground turkey on the palm of your hand, and then place a spoonful of the cheese and onion mixture on the center. Ball up the turkey meat to cover the cheese and onion, and then lightly flatten to form a patty. Repeat for the remaining turkey and cheese and onion mixture.
Heat the olive oil in a pan over medium heat, then cook the patties one at a time. Each side should take about 2-3mins. each.
Serve and enjoy!

Sweet and Sour Turkey Stir-Fry

You don't always hear of a turkey stir-fry, but why not? This dish is delicious, healthy, and brings a twist to stir-fry dishes.

Samantha Michaels

Ingredients:

¼ lb. Lean Ground Turkey
½ Onion, minced
¼ Red Bell Pepper, diced
½ Red Apple, diced
½ teaspoon cinnamon
½ teaspoon Lemon Juice
3 tablespoons Sugar-free Strawberry Jam
1 tablespoon Olive Oil

Procedure:

Heat 1 tablespoon of olive oil in a pan over medium heat.
Sauté the onions, red bell peppers and apple just until the onions are soft and translucent.
Add the lean turkey, season with cinnamon and lemon juice, and then add the fat-free strawberry jam.
Sauté until the turkey is cooked.
Transfer to plate and enjoy.

Turkey Meatballs

Turkey can be just as good as other meats but much healthier. This recipe allows you to enjoy classic favourite, meatballs, and do so with the healthy twist of turkey meat.

Ingredients:

1 lb. Ground Turkey
½ teaspoon Oregano
½ teaspoon Basil
½ teaspoon Garlic, minced
½ teaspoon Parsley
1 Egg
3 oz. Tomato Sauce

¼ cup Parmesan Cheese
¼ cup Green Pepper, diced
1 Onion, diced
2 tablespoons Olive Oil

Procedure:

Place all the ingredients except the olive oil in a bowl and mix it all together to create a uniform mixture.
Measure out 1 tablespoon of the mixture and form into a ball. Do with the rest of the mixture.
Heat the olive oil in a non-stick pan over medium heat. When the oil is hot, place the turkey meatballs in the pan and cook for about 15minutes, or until the outside is browned and crispy. Make sure that the turkey is cooked all the way through.
Serve and enjoy!

Turkey Meatloaf

This recipe is very easy to do but packs very strong flavors. It can be made ahead of time or can be stored in the refrigerator after cooking for future use.

Ingredients:

1 lb. Ground Turkey
2 tablespoons Worcestershire Sauce
1 Onion, diced
½ teaspoon Salt
¼ teaspoon Garlic Powder
½ teaspoon Sage
¼ cup Low fat Blue Cheese
½ teaspoon Pepper

Procedure:

Samantha Michaels

Combine all the ingredients in a bowl and mix together until you have a uniform blend.

Shape into a loaf and place on an oven-safe dish.

Pre-heat the oven to 350°F.

Bake the turkey meatloaf for 1 hour or until the meat is browned and cooked through.

Serve and enjoy.

CHAPTER 4- MAIN ENTREES- FISH DISHES

Baked Tilapia

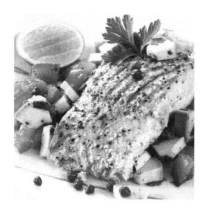

Many people like to cook tilapia because it is quite easy to prepare and it is known for absorbing flavours very well. One healthy way to serve it is by baking it in the oven.

Ingredients:

4 pcs. tilapia fillets, measuring approximately 1.5 lbs. in total
2 tbsp. lemon juice (around 30 mL)
1 tbsp. virgin olive oil
2 tsp. oregano
½ tsp. paprika
1 tbsp. freshly chopped parsley
Salt and pepper to taste
¼ cup Parmesan cheese, grated (optional)

Procedure:

Pre-heat your oven to 400°F.

Prepare a flat baking sheet and cover it with parchment paper. You could apply non-stick cooking spray on the baking sheet or you could use aluminum foil if you don't have any parchment paper at home. Make sure the aluminum foil is of high quality so that the lemon juice will not react with it.

Rinse and clean the tilapia fillets in cool, running water. When you're done, dry the fillets by patting them using clean paper towels.

Using a small bowl, mix the virgin olive oil and the lemon juice. Stir well. If you prefer a stronger lemon taste, you may choose to add up to 2 more tbsps. of lemon juice to this recipe.

Add the oregano, paprika, parsley, salt, and pepper to your lemon and virgin oil mixture.

Put the fillets on the baking sheet, making sure that they are evenly spaced apart.

Pour the combined lemon mixture over the fillets. Use a brush to make sure that the mixture is well-absorbed by all parts of the tilapia.8. You can now bake the fillets. At 400°F, it should be done in about 15 minutes or so. One way to know is if the tilapia has already turned completely white or if you can already be flaked evenly with a fork.

(Optional) You can also add grated Parmesan cheese to your tilapia fillets on the last 10 minutes of your baking time if you like.

Serve warm. Enjoy!

Broiled Halibut Fillets

The halibut has little oil and fat content and it is known for absorbing different flavours quite well. This fish tastes really good when you pair it with lemon and garlic.

Ingredients:

4 pcs. halibut fillets, measuring approximately 6 to 8 ounces each
3 tbsp. olive oil

3 cloves garlic, minced
2 tbsp. lemon juice
½ tsp. dried basil
1 tbsp. parsley, freshly chopped
Salt and pepper
Lemon slices and parsley leaves (optional)

Procedure:

Place halibut fillets on a greased baking sheet. Add salt and pepper. Combine the olive oil, garlic, basil, and parsley in a saucepan. Keep the heat low. Heat the ingredients until the margarine has melted and the garlic has browned and softened.
Pour the mixture over the fillets. Make sure that all parts of the fish are well-coated by the mixture.
Heat the broiler and broil the fillets for approximately 10 minutes. During this time period, make sure to turn the fillets at least once.
Test with a fork to see if it's already done. It will flake away easily when you pierce it with a fork.6. Transfer cooked halibut on a plate. You may choose to garnish it with lemon slices and parsley leaves. Enjoy!

Baked Cajun Catfish

Aside from being a diabetic-friendly dish, the baked Cajun catfish gets a lot of compliments from visitors especially when the recipe is done to perfection!

Ingredients:

4 pcs. catfish fillets weighing approximately 8 ounces each
2 tbsp. olive oil
2 tsp. garlic salt
2 tsp. paprika
2 tsp. dried thyme
½ tsp. cayenne pepper

½ tsp. hot pepper sauce
¼ tsp. pepper powder

Procedure:

Using a small bowl, combine the olive oil, garlic salt, paprika, dried thyme, cayenne pepper, hot pepper sauce, and pepper powder. Mix thoroughly.
Brush the mixture over the fillets. Make sure you coat both sides.
Prepare a baking sheet and coat it with a cooking spray. Place fish on the baking sheet and bake the fillets at 450°F.
It should be done in 10 to 13 minutes. You can see it's done if you can already flake it easily with a fork.
Transfer on a plate and serve warm. Enjoy!

Poached Salmon

The poached salmon is a favourite among many because it is quite easy to prepare. In addition, it also doesn't make your house reek of fish after cooking and well, it's truly delicious! It's simply a good meal to serve to friends and family, whatever the occasion is.

Ingredients:

6 pcs. salmon fillets, measuring about 0.5 inches thick and weighing approximately 5 ounces each
2 cups dry white wine
2 cups water
6 peppercorns
1 pc. lemon, sliced
2 tbsp. fresh dill weed
1 celery stalk, chopped finely
1 pc. onion, sliced
Salt to taste

Procedure:

Sprinkle a little salt on the salmon fillets.

On a large skillet, combine the white wine, water, peppercorns, lemon, dill, celery, and onion. Bring the combined ingredients to a boil. Cover the skillet and let it simmer on medium heat for around 10 minutes.

Place the salmon fillets on the skillet. Cook the salmon for 5 to 10 minutes. The cooking time will depend on the fillet's thickness, so you can check if it is done by seeing if it already flakes easily when pierced with a fork. Be careful not to overcook.

Transfer on a plate. Serve and enjoy!

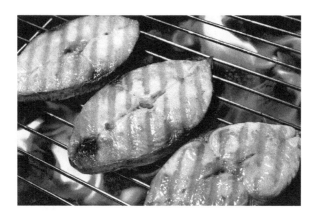

Baked Salmon

Salmon is a real treat to have whether you are on a diet or not. It is packed with omega-3, has healthy proteins and amino acids, and is fairly easy to cook. This recipe calls for a marinade, so it requires a bit of time for the salmon to absorb the flavours. Alternately, you can prepare this ahead of time and just take it out when ready to cook.

Ingredients:

2 cloves, Garlic, minced
1-2 tablespoons Light Olive Oil
1 teaspoon Dried Basil

1 teaspoon Salt

½ teaspoon ground Black Pepper

1 tablespoon Lemon Juice

1 tablespoon fresh Parsley, chopped

2 (6ounce) Salmon Fillets

Procedure:

Prepare the marinade by mixing the minced garlic, olive oil, dried basil, salt, pepper, lemon juice, and parsley in a Ziploc bag.

Place the salmon fillets into the Ziploc bag with the marinade. Refrigerate for at least an hour, making sure that all parts of the salmon are marinated well.

Pre-heat the oven to 375°F or 190°C.

Prepare an oven-safe dish.

When the salmon has been marinated, place over aluminium foil. Pour in the marinade to cover the salmon, and seal the foil.

Place the sealed salmon in the oven-safe dish and bake for 35-45minutes or until the meat is easily flaked with a fork.

Remove from oven. Enjoy.

Sesame-Crusted Tilapia

Another healthy way of serving tilapia is by baking it and infusing the fish with sesame oil flavours. Although it can be marinated 30 minutes before you plan to cook it, it is also recommended to marinate it overnight to let the flavours fully seep in.

Ingredients:

4 pcs. tilapia fillets, weighing around 6 ounces each

2 tbsp. lemon juice

2 tbsp. soy sauce (low sodium)

2 tbsp. ginger, minced

4 tsp. olive oil, divided

1 tsp. sesame oil, divided

2 tbsp. sesame seeds

1/3 cup chicken broth (low sodium)

3 cups green beans, approximately 12 ounces

1/8 tsp. salt

1/8 tsp. ground pepper

Procedure:

Pre-heat your oven to 425°F.

Using a small bowl, combine the lemon juice, soy sauce, 1 tbsp. ginger, 2 tsp. olive oil, and ½ tsp. sesame oil.

Prepare a flat baking sheet, lining it with a parchment paper or high quality aluminium foil. Place the tilapia fillets on the baking sheet, and coat them with lemon juice mixture.

Sprinkle the sesame seeds on the fillets evenly. Bake for about 8 minutes or until the tilapias flake easily.

While you're waiting for the tilapia to cook, heat 2 tsp. olive oil in a non-stick skillet over medium heat. Then, add the remaining ginger and sauté for 1 minute or until it smells good. Add the broth, beans, salt, and pepper. Cover the skillet and let it cook for 5 minutes, or until the beans turn bright green.

When done, turn off the stove and add ½ tsp. sesame oil. Mix well.

When the tilapia is ready use a heat-proof spatula to transfer it onto a serving plate. Divide the green beans evenly among your guests. Enjoy!

Tilapia with Stewed Tomatoes and Spinach

There are many ways to cook tilapia, and if you are looking for a good side dish, spinach and stewed tomatoes would be perfect. This is a low-sodium dish that is easy to prepare, and you will surely score high on your guests because of its delicious taste and health benefits.

Ingredients:

Samantha Michaels

4 pcs. tilapia fillets, approximately 6 to 8 ounces each
12 oz. whole canned tomatoes
4 mushrooms, sliced
½ pc. white onion, sliced
2 cloves of garlic
1 tsp. olive oil
Spinach

Procedure:

In a frying pan, cook the onions using the olive oil. Add the mushroom and garlic and sauté until brown.
Add the canned tomatoes. Cook until it simmers.
Add the tilapia to the pan. Cook it for at least 3 minutes per side.
Put the spinach on top of the tilapia. Cover the pan and cook until the spinach wilts.
When the tilapia is cooked, transfer onto a plate and serve. Enjoy!

Tuna Burger

If you are looking for a healthy alternative to beef burgers, then the tuna fish burger is a highly recommended recipe. It has a lower fat content yet it doesn't compromise flavour.

Ingredients:

200 g tinned tuna in water, drained
60 mL teriyaki sauce
50 g breadcrumbs
1 egg white
¼ tsp. black pepper, ground
¼ tsp. garlic, minced
¼ tsp. hot pepper sauce
¼ tsp. olive oil

Procedure:

In a bowl, mix the tuna, breadcrumbs, teriyaki sauce, and egg whites until all of them are well combined. Make sure all ingredients can be rolled into a ball, with no large pieces of tuna remaining.

Add the black pepper, garlic, and hot pepper sauce to the mixture. Mix thoroughly until the condiments seem evenly distributed. Form two patties afterwards.

In a frying pan, heat the olive oil over medium heat. Cook burgers for about 2 minutes each side, or until both sides are brown enough.

If you wish to make a sandwich, throw in some burger breads, lettuce, tomatoes, and cheese and you're good to go!

Tuna Salad

This tuna salad is very easy to prepare, healthy and tasty to boot as well. It makes an excellent snack on its own, but it can also be used as a sandwich filling. It goes really well with bread or crackers.

Ingredients:

200 g tinned tuna in water, flaked and drained
6 tbsp. salad dressing or mayonnaise
1 tbsp. grated Parmesan cheese
3 tbsp. sweet pickles
1/8 tsp. dried onion flakes
1 tbsp. dried parsley
1 tsp. dried dill
1 pinch garlic granules
¼ tsp. curry powder

Procedure:

In a medium-sized bowl, combine the tuna, mayonnaise or salad dressing, grated Parmesan cheese, and onion flakes. Mix thoroughly.

Season the combined ingredients with parsley, dill, curry powder, and garlic granules.

Use it as a sandwich filling or you can add bread or crackers as sides. Alternatively, you may choose to crush the crackers and mix it with the rest of the ingredients.

Serve and enjoy!

Salmon Burger

Aside from tuna, you can also make healthy burgers out of salmons. Combining it with herbs, breadcrumbs, and seasonings makes it an enjoyable afternoon snack or a light dinner. You may choose to make a sandwich or eat it with a salad on the side.

Ingredients:

450 g tinned salmon, flaked and drained
2 eggs
4 tbsp. fresh parsley, finely chopped
2 tbsp. onion, finely chopped
4 tbsp. breadcrumbs, seasoned dry
2 tbsp. lemon juice
½ tsp. dried basil
1 pinch chillies, crushed
1 tbsp. olive oil
For the sauce:
2 tbsp. light mayonnaise
1 tbsp. lemon juice
1 pinch dried basil

Procedure:

In a medium-sized bowl, combine the salmon, eggs, onion, parsley, 2 tbsp. lemon juice, ½ tsp. basil, crushed chillies, and breadcrumbs. Mix thoroughly and form 6 pcs. burger patties measuring approximate 1.25 cm in thickness.

In a large frying pan, heat the olive oil over medium heat. Once the oil is hot enough, add the salmon burger patties and cook for about 4 minutes each side or until browned.

Mix the mayonnaise, 1 tbsp. lemon juice, and the basil on a small bowl. Spread on the burger patties. Serve and enjoy!

Ginger Lime Salmon

The ginger and lime salmon recipe is relatively easy to prepare and cook but it is still very tasty and appetizing. One of the best things about salmon is it can withstand and hold strong flavours really well. You can grill it or broil it, either way it will turn out great!

Ingredients:

2 pcs. salmon fillet, about 6 ounces each
Mixed peppers, ringed and sliced
Onion rings
Marinade:
½ cup lime juice
1 tsp. fresh ginger, minced
½ tsp. garlic puree
1 tbsp. honey

Procedure:

Mix the ingredients for the marinade.
Put the salmon into the marinade mixture. Let it sit for a few hours. If you have plenty of time, you may want to do it overnight so the marinade will seep well into the salmon.
When the marinated salmon is ready to be cooked, pre-heat your oven to 425°F.
Fill the baking sheet with onion rings and mixed peppers. Place the salmon on top and pour the marinade.
Bake for approximately 20 to 25 minutes or until the salmon flakes easily with a fork. Serve warm and enjoy!

Samantha Michaels

Mediterranean Fish Foil Pockets

This recipe gives you the opportunity to choose from a variety of fishes. Whatever you choose, your meal will surely come out healthy and tasty.

Ingredients:

1 lb. fish fillets, cut to 2 equal parts (cod, tuna, tilapia, or halibut)
2 tbsp. lemon juice
¼ cup black or kalamata olives, coarsely chopped and pitted
1 tbsp. fresh oregano, chopped
1 tbsp. extra-virgin olive oil
1 tbsp. capers, rinsed
½ tsp. ground pepper
½ tsp. salt, divided

Procedure:

Pre-heat your oven to 425°F.
Using a small bowl, combine the lemon juice, olives, oregano, olive oil, and capers.
Creating the foil pocket: Lay 2 sheets of foil on top of each other, measuring around 20 inches each. Coat the top layer with cooking spray, and then put one part of the fish at the centre of the foil. Add the salt and pepper, and then coat with the olive mixture you set aside earlier.
Bring the foil's short ends together. Make sure you leave enough room to get the food steamed and cooked. Fold the foil and seal with a pinch. The seams must be sealed tightly so that the steam will not escape.
Bake the foil pockets in your oven for around 20 minutes or so.
Be careful when you take the foil out of the oven as it is very hot. Open the foil pocket to let the steam escape. Transfer the fish to a plate using a heat-proof spatula. Serve and enjoy!

Fish Gyros with Tzatziki Sauce

If you are looking for a healthy and yet heavy snack, you can't go wrong with fish gyros with tzatziki sauce. This recipe gives you an exciting and easy way to experiment with fish, yogurt, and herbs as main ingredients.

Ingredients:

1 lb. cod or tilapia fillets
4 leaves Boston lettuce
1 clove garlic, minced
¼ tsp. crushed red pepper
¼ cup cilantro, fresh and minced
Salt, pepper, coriander (ground), to taste

Tzatziki Sauce:

2 cups non-fat plain yogurt
1 medium-sized cucumber, seeded, peeled, shredded, and squeezed dry
2 cloves garlic, minced
1 tbsp. extra-virgin olive oil
1 tbsp. red wine vinegar
1 tbsp. fresh thyme (alternatively, 1 ½ tsp. dried thyme)
2 tsp. lemon juice
¼ tsp. salt

Procedure for the Sauce:

Combine all the sauce ingredients in a bowl.
Transfer in a container with a cover and refrigerate for one hour. If you have time, you can let it sit overnight.

Procedure for the Fish Gyros:

Pre-heat your oven to 375°F.2. Season the fish fillets with garlic, red pepper, cilantro, salt, and coriander. Bake for approximately 10 minutes or until the fish flakes easily.

Lay a large leaf of Boston lettuce on a plate. Transfer the fish onto the plate and pour over the tzatziki sauce. Serve warm and enjoy!

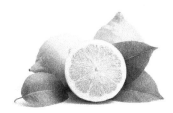

Lemon and Dill Salmon

The lemon and dill salmon is a favourite among many home cooking enthusiasts because it only takes a few ingredients and a little time to cook and prepare. You can also your favourite herbs and capers to add a personal touch to this simple recipe.

Ingredients:

1 lb. wild salmon fillets
1 pc. lemon
1 tsp. dill
Olive oil
Salt and pepper, to taste

Procedure:
Pre-heat your oven to 375°F.
Prepare your baking sheet and line with parchment paper or high quality aluminum foil.
Lay salmon on the baking sheet. Lightly coat the fillets with olive oil. Sprinkle evenly with salt, pepper and dill.
Slice the lemon into thin pieces and place it on top of the salmon.

Bake it for about 20 minutes or until the salmon can be easily flaked. Serve with your favourite vegetables on the side. Enjoy!

Seasoned Tilapia

Many people like cooking the tilapia because you can basically do a lot of things with it. Another easy recipe for this fish is the seasoned tilapia, which only requires you to have some of the most commonly used condiments in the kitchen. In addition to the tilapia, of course!

Ingredients:

4 pcs. tilapia fillets
1 tbsp. extra-virgin olive oil
3 cloves garlic, minced
1 tsp. ginger
1 tsp. paprika
1 tsp. black pepper, ground
1 tsp. dried mustard
1 tsp. oregano
1 tsp. chilli powder
1 pinch cayenne pepper

Procedure:

Pre-heat your oven to 400°F.
Prepare a flat baking sheet and line it with parchment paper.
Combine the paprika, ginger, ground black pepper, dried mustard, oregano, chilli powder, and cayenne pepper in a medium-sized bowl.
Coat each fillet lightly with olive oil. Sprinkle the combined seasonings and garlic and place the fish on the baking sheet.
Bake for about 10 minutes or until the salmon flakes easily. Serve and enjoy!

CHAPTER 5- SNACKS

Buffalo Chicken Tenders

This is an easy recipe for an all-time favourite.

Ingredients:

1 lb. Chicken Breasts
2 tablespoons Olive Oil
¼ cup Hot Sauce

Procedure:

Cut the chicken breasts into strips.
Combine the olive oil and the hot sauce in a zip lock bag, then add the chicken strips and let it marinate for at least 30minutes.
Pre-heat oven to 375°F.
Place the chicken strips in an oven-safe dish and pour remaining marinade over the pieces.
Bake in the pre-heated oven for 12-16 minutes or until cooked through.
Serve and enjoy!

If you are in a hurry, you can just let it marinate for however long you can wait, then cook immediately. Longer marinating time only allows the chicken to absorb more of the heat from the hot sauce. You can serve this with more hot sauce or some celery sticks on the side.

Cauliflower Popcorn

Whoever said that healthy ingredients cannot be eaten as snacks? Here is a simple and healthy 'popcorn' recipe to make you think otherwise.

Ingredients:

1 head Cauliflower
4 tablespoons Olive Oil
1 teaspoon Salt

Procedure:

Pre-heat the oven to 425°F.
Remove the stem from the cauliflower and cut the heads into individual pieces the size of ping-pong balls. Be careful not to cut them too small.
Combine the olive oil and the salt in a large bowl, then whisk together.
Toss in the cauliflower heads into the olive oil and mix to coat all of the pieces.
Transfer the cauliflower onto an oven-safe dish and bake in the pre-heated oven for about 1hour. Make sure to turn the pieces over from time to time to let it cook on all sides.
Serve immediately and enjoy!

You can also add fat-free parmesan cheese, garlic powder, or any seasoning of your choice for an added flavour.

Chicken Lettuce Wraps

Even if you are on a diet, you can enjoy tasty snacks like these chicken lettuce wraps. You can even prepare this ahead of time and serve to guests or family and friends.

Ingredients:

1 Chicken Breast
1 Scallion, diced
½ cup Red Grapes, chopped
2 tablespoons Celery, chopped
1 tablespoon Olive Oil
Salt and Pepper to taste
1 pack Iceberg Lettuce Leaves

Procedure:

Bake the chicken breasts for about 30minutes in 350°F or until cooked through.
Cut the chicken breasts into small cubes.
In a bowl, combine the diced scallions, chopped grapes, celery, olive oil, and salt and pepper, then add the chicken pieces.
Refrigerate until chilled.
To serve, take one lettuce leaf at a time, spoon the chicken mixture into the center, then wrap the lettuce around the chicken mixture. Enjoy!

Egg Salad Wraps

Just because Cycle 1 does not allow you to eat bread does not mean you can no longer enjoy your favourite sandwich recipes. Here is a classic egg sandwich with lettuce leaves instead of bread. Yummy and healthy!

Ingredients:

2 Eggs, hardboiled
Salt and Pepper to taste
2 tablespoons Fat-free Yogurt
Lettuce Leaves

Procedure:

Take the hardboiled eggs and mash them up with a fork.

Add the mayonnaise, and then sprinkle with salt and pepper. Mix everything properly.

When ready to eat, get a lettuce leaf, place a spoonful of the egg mixture in the middle, then wrap the lettuce around the egg.

Enjoy!

If the yogurt is too strong for you, you can simply substitute with some olive oil and a dash of vinegar.

Mock Mashed Potatoes

If you find yourself craving for mashed potatoes, try this recipe out so that you still stick to your diet. Enjoy!

Ingredients:

1 head Cauliflower
2 tablespoons Non-fat Yogurt
¼ teaspoon Garlic Powder
¼ teaspoon Onion Powder
¼ teaspoon Salt

Procedure:

Remove the hard stem of the cauliflower and cut into smaller pieces.

Steam the cauliflower until very soft.

Mash the cauliflower, and then add the yogurt and the seasonings.

Mix well and enjoy!

You can also use your favourite seasonings or adjust to your preferred taste.

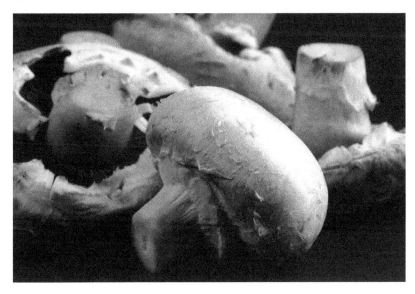

Stuffed Mushrooms

Stuffed mushrooms are great snacks that are both filling and delicious. The best thing about this recipe is that it lets you keep on course with your diet while still letting you enjoy flavourful snacks.

Ingredients:

1 lb. Whole Mushrooms
2 pcs. Tomatoes, diced
½ cup Ground Turkey
Salt and Pepper to taste
¼ cup Fat-free Mozzarella or Parmesan Cheese

Procedure:

Pre-heat oven to 350°F.
Clean the whole mushrooms and remove the middle.
In a bowl, mix together the ground turkey and the diced tomatoes.
Season with salt and pepper.

Stuff the mushrooms with the ground turkey mixture and place on an oven-safe dish.

Top the stuffed mushrooms with mozzarella or parmesan cheese, then bake in the pre-heated oven for 15-20minutes or until the mushrooms have softened and the cheese begins to brown.

Serve and enjoy!